CR
AND COLITIS

A Whole Foods Plant-Based Approach

EDWARD ESKO
ALEX JACK
VIRGINIA HARPER

Foreword by Sommer White, M.D.

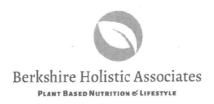

Berkshire Holistic Associates

PLANT BASED NUTRITION & LIFESTYLE

Published by Berkshire Holistic Associates
A division of Planetary Health, Inc.
P.O. Box 487
Becket, Mass. 01223
BerkshireHolistic.com
Published in Association with the International Macrobiotic Institute

ISBN-13: 9798615718380
ISBN-10: 1535197218

Previously published as *Crohn's and Colitis: The Macrobiotic Approach*

Whereas chimpanzees spend five hours a day chewing raw food, a single hour suffices for people eating cooked food. The advent of cooking enabled humans to eat more kinds of food, to devote less time to eating, and to make do with smaller teeth and shorter intestines.

YUVAL NOAH HARARI, *SAPIENS: A BRIEF HISTORY OF HUMANKIND*

Contents

———

FOREWORD

We are entering an exciting new period in healthcare where holistic practices are being integrated with western medicine. Current trends are moving away from the limiting symptoms-based approach of diagnosis and treatment to an encompassing patient-centered approach. Plagued by unanswered questions and unsuccessful treatments that can lead to other issues, such as unwanted side effects and dependency, western physicians and patients are looking for ways to address all aspects of illness including the root cause.

In addition, each day more physicians and patients are acknowledging the impact food and lifestyle has on the development of illness. New scientific studies repeatedly reveal the benefits of eating a primarily plant-based diet, and the field of epigenetics has shown how food, meditation and lifestyle affect gene expression. Mind, body and spirit all play a role in wellness, and these factors impact sickness and health to a much larger degree than once believed. Management and treatment have begun to focus on a comprehensive approach using multiple healing modalities.

As an Emergency Medicine physician practicing in a busy Los Angeles Emergency Department, I was the epitome of a focused, fast-paced doctor who was trying to thrive in a broken system. Following strict algorithms for medical management and adhering to impersonal governmental and hospital regulations led me to a path of Band-Aid management and symptom control.

With a computer in hand, and its list of past medical histories, medications and surgeries, there was little need for personal interaction. And with less personal interaction, came dissatisfaction, a lack of fulfillment, as well as a realization of ineffectiveness.

However, when my focus began to shift away from this method and instead toward the person in front of me, my practice and view of medicine began to radically change. This experience mirrored my own struggle with chronic fatigue and recurrent infections.

It was during this critical time in my life that I turned to macrobiotics in order to heal myself and find explanations and solutions that western medicine couldn't provide. I began studying about food and food preparation, energetic connections, yin and yang, the five transformations, chakras and meridians. I started to look differently at illness and the human body. Applying concepts of yin and yang to western medicine became not only fascinating, but also extremely helpful in understanding what was occurring with my patients.

Macrobiotics provides a foundation for diagnosing and treating illness, as well as explanations for why people have conditions and how they can overcome them. It identifies the constitution, or genetic predisposition of a person, as well as the current condition. Tools such as visual diagnosis are used that lead to a deeper understanding and connection with the patient. Macrobiotics also emphasizes that healers use intuition to guide their patients to health, and it teaches the importance of healing from within as well as the steps to do so.

When I started studying macrobiotics, I had no idea that it would become a pillar for my Integrative Medicine practice. Now as I consistently incorporate its principles into my personal and professional life, I understand the journey of personal commitment and self-care, as well as the challenges and excitement in achieving optimal health.

Macrobiotic teachings illustrate the importance of acknowledging and balancing all aspects in order to attain true health and maintain freedom from illness. Offering clear explanations to the pathologic development of disease, they illustrate how when we look deeper at energetics and connections, we see the whole picture and can then direct a person to a path of innate, authentic healing.

The teachings of macrobiotics illustrate the crucial roles of both practitioners and patients in transforming the current medical system. While presenting explanations beyond the realm of rigid scientific theory—where information can often be confusing, conflicting, and misleading—the macrobiotic perspective imparts a clear understanding of illness. It emphasizes the importance of taking our health into our own hands and how the empowerment of doing so will facilitate and support us on a journey of positive healing.

Sommer White, M.D.
Vitality Medical Center

Studies show that red meat intake is associated with higher levels of inflammatory markers like c-reactive protein (CRP), even when controlling for other dietary and lifestyle factors. Meanwhile, a high intake of whole grains reduces CRP.

GOOGLE

PREFACE

My days of confusion, pain, and suffering are a mere memory. Who would have known that the seven long years of suffering with inflammatory bowel disease labeled as Crohn's would become the catalyst for health and wellness in my life. Now, thirty-five years later, I look back with heartfelt gratitude at the healing journey through which I acquired the knowledge and practice to claim a Crohn's-free life!

It all began with the information you are about to read in this book. The macrobiotic way of healing became my road to freedom from Crohn's disease. A freedom acquired through learning and practicing the fundamental principles of the lifestyle that helped me become self-directed in my health. This kind of knowledge gives you the hope to take control and self-navigate with care and consistency through the maze of scary diagnoses and stifling medical protocols.

It is with great pleasure and enthusiasm that I collaborate in this writing. I will share experiences, recipes, and therapies that helped me to heal and that have been effective with the thousands of people that I've been privileged to guide as an author and a macrobiotic counselor. My personal counseling practice has given me firsthand knowledge and experience in dealing with the effects of inflammation within the body. Inflammation is the root cause of digestive breakdown and autoimmune conditions. My mode of operandi is the macrobiotic philosophy. It is from this viewpoint—the yin/yang understanding of balance—that I derive my analysis and protocols for clients.

The goal in my practice is to help people free themselves from pain while learning to utilize these principles in becoming self-aware and responsible for their well being. Only from this vantage point can a disease-free life be obtained.

To unlock the secret behind the macrobiotic approach is to discover a way of life and lifestyle which drives our mental and physical well-being, bringing restorative and regenerative energies to create harmony and balance, peace and hope, within each of us. It was our great teacher Michio Kushi who said, "Peace begins in the kitchen and the pantries, gardens and backyards, where food is grown and prepared. The energies of nature and the infinite universe are absorbed through the foods we eat and transmuted into our thoughts and actions."

By acquiring a strong foundation of the principle of macrobiotics, the reader will be prepared to understand the role of food beyond nutrition while understanding the energetic influence of digesting *everything*. Accordingly, you will learn to identify energetic influence in foods, seasons, and how your body functions.

Virginia Harper
Author *Controlling Crohn's the Natural Way*

Digestion, of all the bodily functions, is the one which
exercises the greatest influence on the mental state
of an individual.
JEAN-ANTHELME BRILLAT-SAVARIN (1755-1826)

Definitions*

Yin

The primary expansive force of the universe producing upward movement, lightness, an outside position, water and air, the colors green and blue, and the world of plants.

Yang

The primary contractive force of the universe producing downward movement, heaviness, an inside position, solid matter, the colors brown and red, and the world of animals.

*Note: The terms "yin" and "yang" are Chinese in origin. Any terms that describe complementary/opposites may be used in their place.

CROHN'S AND COLITIS

Edward Esko

To understand Crohn's, colitis, and other inflammatory bowel syndromes (IBS) let us see the digestive system in terms of yin and yang. The first thing we do is to classify the digestive system into upper and lower. The upper portion includes the mouth, the esophagus, and the upper stomach. The lower portion includes the lower stomach, the duodenum, the small intestine and large intestine. The upper region is more yin or expansive while the lower region is more yang or contractive.

Not only do we have up and down, we also have left and right. This is most relevant when we look at the colon. The colon extends across both sides of the body. On the right side we have the ascending colon, on the left, the descending colon. Which side is more yin and which side is more yang? Which direction is energy moving on the right side? Up. Here we have the ascending colon, more yin. Which direction is energy moving on the left side? Down. Here we have the descending colon, more yang. The rectum, muscular and contracting, is the most yang.

Next we can see the acid and alkaline balance of the digestive system. Generally, acid is more yin and alkaline more yang. What is the primary digestive secretion in the mouth? Alkaline saliva. That is why chewing is so important to make our food more alkaline. The next part of the digestive system, the stomach, secretes strong acid, which is yin. If food is properly mixed with saliva in the mouth, the proper acid secretion occurs in the stomach.

Next is the duodenum. The duodenum is the connector between the stomach and the small intestine. The duodenum receives from the liver and pancreas very strong alkaline secretions. The duodenum receives bile from the liver and pancreatic juice from the pancreas. The small intestine produces a more acid secretion, while the large intestine produces a more alkaline environment.

If we eat foods that support our digestive tract, digestive harmony proceeds day to day without any problem. What foods support our digestive harmony? Which foods are good and which are harmful? Let's look at the teeth. We have twenty molars and premolars. The word "molar" means "millstone." Millstones are used for crushing wheat or other grains and fibers into flour. These teeth are used for crushing grains, beans, and seeds, and are not tearing teeth. We have eight incisors. These are cutting teeth. These are the teeth of deer or rabbits that come into your garden and eat your vegetables. That means twenty-eight grain and vegetable teeth versus four canine teeth. What is the ratio here? The ratio is seven to one. Yes animal food can be eaten but much less than plant food. Everyone is now recommending a plant-based diet. Macrobiotics was advocating such since the 1950s in Europe and America.

Another reason for a plant-based diet is the structure of the digestive system as a whole. Carnivores have short digestive tracts. Ours is much longer. Which part is shorter in the carnivore? The colon. Why is that? Ours is about five feet squeezed in. When prey is killed, like the gazelle being taken down by the lion, what happens in the body of the lion in the African heat? The meat immediately starts to break down and decompose. It decomposes into toxic bacteria and toxic protein compounds like ammonia.

It is important for decomposing flesh to be rapidly discharged from the body of the lion. Our digestive system is much longer. So when we eat meat, especially in the hot summer, there is plenty of opportunity for decomposition and trouble to begin. That is why in modern America, which is still a meat-eating culture, we see so many problems caused by meat and animal food eating and a lack of plant fiber.

By the way, how is our digestive tract different from that of plant-eating animals such as cows or sheep? Their digestive systems are longer and they have several stomachs. Why? It is very hard to break down tough raw plant fiber or cellulose. They have to chew all day long. What a life. No worries or cares. Because they spend all day chewing they have no time to paint the Mona Lisa, fly in the space shuttle, or invent the smart phone. Their life is very limited. It was fire and cooking that liberated us from that kind of life. It made our free life possible.

The macrobiotic diet is the ideal ratio between plant and animal food. It suggests an ideal ratio of grain to vegetable.

It is the ideal utilization of plant protein, for example beans or soy products together with grain. It also recommends the use of naturally fermented foods. With this ideal pattern, combined with proper chewing, digestive problems are rare. Unfortunately, that is often not the case. Let us see how dietary imbalances cause problems in the digestive system. Where does a heavy meat and animal food diet cause trouble? Does trouble arise in the yin, upper part or the yang, lower part? It tends to arise in the lower digestive tract. If we eat extreme yin food, refined sugar, tropical fruit, and strong spice, trouble tends to arise in the upper digestive tract. Moreover, these extremes tend to exacerbate inflammation in the digestive system as a whole.

A related example of extreme yang causing trouble in the more yang parts of the body arises from eating too many eggs. Eggs often negatively affect the ovaries, which are yang. To confirm this, Google "balut." Balut is a delicacy in the Philippines. It is a fertilized duck egg that is allowed to mature. Right before hatching, the egg is hard-boiled. When they peel off the shell, there is a duck embryo inside which they eat. I saw this on my favorite TV show, *Bizarre Foods*, on the Travel Channel.

In *Bizarre Foods* the host, Andrew Zimmern, travels around the world eating the most exotic, local, and unusual foods imaginable. He is a very yang guy. He fearlessly eats exotic local foods and thereby bonds with the local people and experiments on himself with a bold, somewhat macrobiotic spirit. The show is highly recommended for all students of macrobiotics.

Compare the image of a "balut" to the image of a "dermoid cyst." A dermoid cyst is a hard cyst that arises in the ovaries. Strangely enough, it resembles the image of a balut, suggesting that consumption of eggs may be the cause. The ovaries are yang and eggs are yang. Why are eggs so yang? What is an egg? It is entire germ of the organism. Once fertilized, it changes into extreme yin, billions of cells proliferate and the complete organism comes into being.

A high meat diet often causes trouble in the lowest portion of the colon, which is the most yang region. A high meat diet often means a diet low in plant fiber. Normally the bowel movement is more bulky because of fiber. When fiber is lacking and plenty of yang animal food is consumed, the stool becomes yang and compact. Blockage or constipation easily occurs. Constipation caused by contraction, or yang animal food, is widespread in our society. Eating meat is the direct cause.

How do we see that condition? Very thin tight lips. I often show a photo of former President George H.W. Bush as an example. His lips were very thin and tight. The reason I did that was that he invited us to "read my lips." So we did. He also mentioned that he hated broccoli, which, like other fiber-rich green vegetables, helps maintain digestive health. Yin constipation is the opposite. A good example is the lips of Angelina Jolie. They are swollen and expanded. Sugar, tropical fruit, and chocolate may be contributing to her condition.

Chronic constipation caused by meat often means that blockage is occurring in the lower colon. Waste material and toxins accumulate there. When a person with this condition needs to go to the toilet, they often are forced to strain. The pressure caused by straining causes a variety of problems. A very common problem is that the veins in the rectum and anus begin to bulge out. That condition is known as hemorrhoids.

Hemorrhoids are very common result of yang blockage in the lower colon. In order to cure hemorrhoids, it is necessary to stop eating animal food and adopt a vegan macrobiotic diet for a time. Fish can be avoided as well. When the hemorrhoids recede, then some white meat or other fish can be eaten. Macrobiotics offers a cure for this common problem.

Another problem occurs when straining causes pockets to blow out in the lower colon. That condition is called "diverticulitis." These pockets often become infected and inflamed. I recently saw a client with this condition. He didn't know that he had it. He was forced to go to the emergency room due to high fever caused by infection. He needed antibiotics to relieve his infection. Then they discovered diverticulitis. People eating a high fiber plant-based diet don't develop this condition. Plant foods don't cause this. Meat causes this.

What is the problem with the way meat is being eaten today? If you watch the Travel Channel you can see very clearly. One popular show is called, *Bacon Nation*. The host travels around the country searching for the best bacon. Another show is called, *Man Versus Food*. The star eats giant grilled steaks without any vegetables or fiber foods. I can't imagine how he is able to survive.

Some of you may remember Campbell's Soup. I remember Campbell's Chicken Noodle Soup. So what was the major complaint? There's no chicken in here. It's mostly noodles and the pieces of chicken are tiny. Or Campbell's Beef and Barley Soup: the beef is cut into tiny little pieces. The soup is mostly barley. I used to feel cheated. How do you compare that way of consuming animal food to today's sixteen-ounce steak? Which is safer, more traditional? Our ancestors ate stew and soup, with lots of fiber. Vegetables, grains, and other foods that counteracted the meat were part of the meal. The amount of meat was minimal.

We have now reviewed the digestive tract as a whole, classifying the different regions into yin and yang. We also know the basic yin and yang of foods, which foods are extreme and which are more centrally balanced. Grains are right in the middle. This is very valuable information. We also know that plant foods are compatible with our digestive structure, and that animal foods can set in motion a whole spectrum of digestive disorders, beginning with constipation and moving through to problems like hemorrhoids and diverticulitis.

Excessive intake of animal food can lead to far more serious conditions. Examples are Crohn's disease and ulcerative colitis. We can see in the illustration how these conditions differ. Although these distinctions are not absolute, ulcerative colitis tends to begin in the lower colon. Crohn's, although it can begin anywhere in the digestive tract, often begins in the ascending colon and small intestine. Which tendency is more yin and which is more yang.

Ulcerative colitis tends to have a more yang cause, while Crohn's tends to have a more yin cause.

Keep in mind that when we say "more yin," we actually are referring to degrees of animal food, and not necessarily yin extremes like sugar or chocolate, although those can contribute to inflammation. We saw that eggs are the most yang, red meat or beef is next, especially processed or grilled meat. What comes after that, going along the spectrum from most yang to least yang? We have eggs, grilled meat, meat, and then poultry, including grilled chicken. Next comes cheese, especially hard salty cheese.

By itself milk is a yin food, although it comes from the yang body of an animal. What is the purpose of mammal milk? Its purpose is to make the newborn grow. Especially large mammals like horses or cows. Human milk is much more sensitive and geared more to brain development. When you filter out the fat and liquid from milk, you're left with more yang protein and minerals. If you age that with salt, you get hard salty cheese. Hard cheese tends to affect the deeper regions of the body like the ovaries and uterus. Cheese has a different effect on the body than soft dairy like milk, yogurt, and cottage cheese. Milk and other soft dairy products tend to affect the upper and more surface regions. These products are increasingly linked to breast conditions, including breast cancer. That is especially true with milk from cows fed growth and other artificial hormones.

From what we've seen so far, what type of animal food do you think would be more associated with colitis that begins in the lower colon? Heavy meat and animal food are often the cause. What foods do you think are more linked with Crohn's? Foods like chicken and cheese, which are less strongly yang, are often triggers. Hard cheese, including that in pizza, would definitely contribute. Hard cheese can also contribute to the development of tumors or polyps in the upper or ascending colon. Once again, as with colitis, extreme yin foods such as chocolate, spices, and sugar accelerate inflammation, as does milk and other dairy foods.

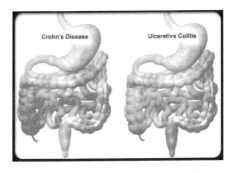

Crohn's disease often begins in the ascending colon and small intestine. Colitis often begins in the lower or descending colon.

Let me illustrate this with two cases I saw recently. One was a forty-year-old man from Houston Texas. When you hear Houston Texas, what red flag appears? Barbecue. He grew up eating plenty of barbecue with lots of hot sauce. What a poor combination. The hot sauce contributes to the inflammation caused by grilled meat. As a result, he developed ulcerative colitis in the lower colon. He went for treatment but didn't change his diet or lifestyle. He kept eating barbecue and hot sauce. Eventually the entire colon became affected. By that time he was having about forty diarrhea episodes per day with blood. (Some patients have up to seventy episodes per day.) Since nothing worked, the doctors told him the only thing they could do was to remove the entire colon.

I consulted with him over Skype. Unfortunately, he had already had the colon removed. He showed many signs of over-consuming fluid. Why do you think he was consuming too much fluid? Because the large intestine's function is to absorb water, so now he had to compensate by taking in lots of fluid. The average time between the beginning of ulcerative colitis in the lower colon and its spread to the entire intestine is about ten years. That gives us an opportunity to intervene with macrobiotics to stop the progression of the colitis and begin to reverse it through diet.

Another case was a man in his mid-forties from New Jersey with Chron's disease. His symptoms were like that of colitis: frequent diarrhea with blood and abdominal pain. His favorite foods were not necessarily beef or barbecue, but chicken and cheese, which are somewhat less yang, and which he ate practically every day for many years.

Colon cancer is the final and potentially terminal stage in the disruption of the digestive tract caused by extreme diet. In America, cancer of the lower digestive tract, especially colorectal cancer, is common. Foods such as grilled steak, hamburger, pulled pork, bacon and other processed meats are often triggers. A food such as a triple bacon cheeseburger makes no sense from the point of view of natural balance. Any one of these items is problematic; the combination of all three is absolutely crazy.

Irritable bowel syndrome, or IBS, has a different cause. It is often a temporary condition caused by the intake of extreme yin such as tropical fruits or spices. People who travel to India, Mexico, or other warm regions may develop it. It is easier to cure than degenerative conditions like Chron's and colitis. One way to prevent it is to eat umeboshi plum, paste, or extract on a daily basis if you travel to these regions.

Together with avoiding the foods that cause trouble in the digestive tract and adopting a plant-based macrobiotic diet, there are several remedies that can help in the recovery from Crohn's, colitis, and other digestive disorders. They include:

Roasted Salt Pack
When someone is having forty or more diarrhea episodes per day, is this over- or under-active energy? This is super active energy. So we need a remedy with the opposite energy: calming, soothing, and contracting. In macrobiotics we have a very effective remedy called the Roasted Salt Pack. (It can also be used to relieve aches or pains anywhere in the body, including in the joints.) To prepare it, roast a cup of sea salt in a dry skillet until it becomes hot. Roasted salt can become very hot, so test it after several minutes to ensure it doesn't become too hot. Roast it in the skillet with a wooden spoon as if you were roasted nuts or seeds, waving the spoon back and forth to ensure even

roasting. Pour the hot salt into a medium-sized towel and tie the ends to form a tight hot bag. Apply directly to the abdomen as you would a hot water bottle. Remove when it cools off. You can reuse the salt four or five times before replacing it with fresh salt. This remedy is very helpful in reducing the inflammation and frequent diarrhea episodes associated with Crohn's, colitis, and inflammatory or irritable bowel syndromes.

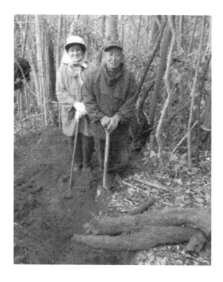

Kuzu root (lower right)

Ume-Sho-Kuzu

The next remedy for over active diarrhea is a big deep root known as kuzu (kudzu). What properties does this deep root have? Kuzu has warming and condensing properties that cause the colon to become firm and tight.

Kuzu causes loose stools to become firm. It also calms overactive energy and reduces inflammation. When combined with natural—not artificial—ume plum or paste, which help alkalize the digestive tract, it is a very effective remedy. Umeboshi also has antibacterial effects. It can be used for Crohn's, colitis, IBS, constipation caused by swollen intestines, and disorders such as acid reflex or stomach ulcer. Ume-Sho-Kuzu is a thick hot tea that can be seasoned with organic shoyu, or soy sauce. It has soothing, calming, and gently alkalizing effects. (Refer to the recipe for Ume-Sho-Kuzu in the *Special Dishes and Remedies* section.)

Over the years I have counseled thousands of people toward recovery from digestive and bowel disorders. One case especially comes to mind. She was a twenty-year-old college student in the Boston area. She had been diagnosed with ulcerative colitis. Her condition was so severe that her Boston doctors were insisting on removal of her colon. Naturally she and her family were in a state of panic. She and her mother came to see me at the Kushi Institute. They were sobbing. They were in despair. I did my best to calm them down and reassure them that there was a way to escape that bleak future.

The way was actually quite simple. She would have to completely change her diet. She would have to stop the foods that were causing her ulcers and inflammation and eat foods that would heal her colon. I recommended a simple macrobiotic diet plus the home remedies noted above (the Roasted Salt Pack and Ume-Sho-Kuzu tea.)

She committed herself to healing and embarked on the macrobiotic recommendations. Six weeks later she visited her doctor for a checkup. The doctor told her that he didn't know how to explain it, but that her condition had improved. In fact it had improved to the point that the operation was not necessary. He told her to keep doing what she had been doing and to come back in several months. This continued for the next year until at one point, the doctor said she was in total remission and could go on with her life.

Another, somewhat well known example is that of Virginia Harper. Virginia was diagnosed at age 23 with Crohn's and given a bleak prognosis. She searched for alternatives and found macrobiotics. Through diligent study and practice, she was able to recover completely and was pronounced, "Crohn's free" by her doctors. She wrote a book about her experience, *Controlling Crohn's Disease: The Natural Way*, now in its fifth edition. She has guided thousands of clients both at her center outside of Nashville and around the world.

Recently, our macrobiotic center invited Virginia Harper to lead a special one-week residential seminar titled *Controlling Crohn's and Colitis* at its campus in the Berkshires. Normally about a dozen students with these conditions attend the seminar. Their stories are often sad and touching since these conditions have such a strongly negative impact on a person's quality of life. However, their experiences with macrobiotics are equally hopeful.

During the seminar, I asked Virginia whether or not the participants had improved during the week. She broke out into a big smile and said that all the men and women who attended her seminar had experienced dramatic improvements in their general wellbeing and quality of life. Many were confident they could recover completely. Through these simple examples, we see that macrobiotics can offer hope to the millions of people around the world suffering from these conditions.

Source: Lecture at the Macrobiotic Summer Conference
Edited by Noreen Dillman

DIET, CROHN'S, AND THE MICROBIOME

Alex Jack

One of the biggest discoveries in modern biology is the *microbiome*. This is defined as the ecological community of bacteria, viruses, fungi, and other microorganisms that dwell in the human gut, skin, mouth, and other parts of the body. Altogether trillions of microbes inhabit our digestive tract and other organs, weigh about 3 pounds, and take up 1-3% of body mass. The intestines alone contain an estimated 40,000 species, and bacterial and other microbial cells in the human body outnumber somatic and germ cells by nearly 10 to 1. The human genome contains about 25,000 genes, about the same size as that of a worm, and half that of rice. But most of the genes in the human body are microbial. Altogether, bacteria and other single-cell beings contain 4.5 million genes, or about 99.5% of the collective genome in the human organism.

Overwhelmingly, these tiny denizens are beneficial. It has long been known that bacteria in the villi of the small intestine assist in the final digestion and assimilation of food. Others can modify the regulation of neurotransmitters, stimulate lymphoid tissue, and assist in the repair of damaged cells. The large intestine also plays a vital role. In addition to absorbing water and storing waste as feces, the colon harbors microbes that synthesize biotin, vitamin K, and other vitamins; synthesize amino acids; and transform bile acid.

The lower G.I. tract also stimulates bacterial growth and produces SCFA (short-chain fatty acids) and other compounds that digest fiber and prevent inflammation. The microflora also lead to the production and release of cytokines, chemokines, and phagocytes that are a part of the body's overall immune function.

Over the last generation, a major nutritional trend involves the consumption of bacteria and other live microorganisms that are beneficial to human health. They are known as *probiotics* and typically involve consuming *Lactobaccilus, Bifodobacterium*, and other strains commercially available as dietary supplements. Traditionally, fermented foods such as miso, shoyu, tempeh, sauerkraut, and yogurt served this function and helped to protect against inflammation, diarrhea, and other bowel troubles, as well as urinary tract infections, high blood pressure and high cholesterol, influenza and other respiratory disorders, and eczema and other skin conditions. Closely connected are *prebiotics* or compounds in selectively fermented fibers (such as the skin of onions, apple peels, and chicory roots) that nourish the beneficial bacteria already in the large intestine.

After more than a century of demonizing "germs," the medical profession is discovering that most microorganisms live symbiotically with human beings and are indispensable to our growth and development. Instead of killing them with antibiotics and antiviral drugs, they should be encouraged, nurtured, and replenished. Research has found that exposing children to microbes may prevent allergies, asthma, and other autoimmune diseases later in life. Instead of compulsive hand washing and use of chemical sanitizer gel, pediatricians are now encouraging kids to play in the dirt, put toys in their mouth, visit local farms, and frolic outdoors with their pets. As Mary Ruebush, a microbiology and immunology instructor, explains in her new book, *Why Dirt Is Good*: "Not only does this allow for 'practice' of immune responses, which will be necessary for protection, but it also plays a critical role in teaching the immature immune response what is best ignored."[1]

Crohn's disease, colitis, gastroenteritis, leaky gut, and other digestive disorders may result from the disruption or imbalance of the microbes in the intestines. In *10% Human: How Your Body's Microbes Hold the Key to Health and Happiness*, British science writer Alana Collen compares the colony of microbes in our bodies to a rainforest. She likens the devastation of microorganisms in the human intestines by chemicals in food and water to the destruction of the South American rainforests. "For the complex ecosystem of the gut, on a scale a million times tinier [than a rainforest], the principles still stand. Antibiotic chainsaws and invasive pathogens pull apart the web of life that's forced a balance through countless subtle interactions. If the destruction is large enough, the system cannot bounce back.

Instead, it collapses. In the rainforest, this is habitat destruction. In the body, it causes *dysbiosis*—an unhealthy balance of microbiota."[2]

Current research shows that the unhealthy imbalance of microbes in the colon may be largely responsible for overweight and obesity; a precursor to many digestive disorders, as well as cardiovascular disease, diabetes, and selected cancers. While fat and sugar are routinely blamed for causing overweight and obesity, excessive consumption of these items in the modern diet does not necessarily lead to weight gain. Countries with higher per capita fat consumption (up to 46% of the diet) have lower BMIs (Body Mass Indexes) than nations with lower fat intakes (as low as 27%). Similarly, sugar consumption doesn't automatically lead to weight gain. The intake of sugar in Australia fell from 30 to 25 teaspoons a day between 1980 and 2003, yet obesity multiplied three times.[3]

A lack of fiber in the diet appears to be the main cause of dysbiosis, or disharmony in the microbiome. In a study comparing children aged 2 to 6 in Burkina Faso and in Florence, Italy, researchers found that the African kids consumed about 6.5 percent of their diet in the form of fiber, while the European youngsters took in only 2 percent. Seventy-five percent of the microbiota in the African children consisted of *Prevotella* and *Xylanibacter*, types of beneficial bacterial that cause enzymes to break down cellulose and other indigestible compounds of plants and strengthen the lining of the intestinal tract.

The Italian kids completely lacked those two strains

and their gut contained primarily *Firmicutes*, a type of bacteria linked to obesity and leaky gut syndrome.[4]

In studies with young Crohn's patients, researchers have found beneficial microbes to be rare and harmful ones flourishing.[5] In another pediatric study, the intestines of Crohn's sufferers showed an abundance of *Enterobacteriaceas, Pasteruellacaea,* and *Fusobacteriaceae* and decreased amounts of *Erysipelotrichales, Bacteroidales,* and *Clostridiales*, a pattern of reduced microbial diversity strongly correlated with disease. Comparisons with Crohn's patients who took antibiotics and those who didn't showed exposure to pharmaceuticals increased the microbial dysbiosis linked to the disorder. "There is now overwhelming evidence that enteric bacteria play a major role in the pathogenesis of Crohn's disease, either as causative agents or mitigating factors," observed Rodrick J. Chiodini, a researcher at Texas Tech University Health Sciences Center.[6] Animal studies have confirmed this link. Healthy mice that received transplanted disease-associated microbiota developed inflammatory bowels. The German team that conducted this experiment reported that the intestinal disorders were not caused by individual strains of bacteria but the overall combination and balance of strains in the gut.[7]

The rapid rise of Crohn's in modern society has been linked to dietary factors, including increased consumption of animal protein, casein (the protein in milk and dairy foods), a higher ratio of omega-6 to omega-3 polyunsaturated fatty acids, and reduced intake of plant protein. To these nutritional factors, the health of the microflora in the body must now be added.

Celiac, another digestive disorder characterized by the inability to digest gluten, has been linked to dysbiosis. Zonulin, a protein produced in the liver and intestines and triggered by harmful bacteria, loosens the chains of the gut lining, leading to an autoimmune response that attacks the cells of the patient's own gut. Beside Celiac, Zonulin is associated with Type 1 diabetes and irritable bowel syndrome (IBS).

"The anatomy of our digestive system, with its emphasis on the large intestine as a home for plant-loving microbes, and a long appendix that acts as a safe-house and storage facility, serves to remind us that we are not pure carnivores, and plants are our staple diet," Alana Collen concludes in *10% Human*. "The nutrient we're missing out on is fiber, but it is plants that we're forgetting to eat. You are what you eat. What's more, you are what *they* eat. With each meal you make, spare a thought for your microbes. What would *they* like you to put in your mouth today?"[8]

As part of a balanced diet, fermented foods like miso, tempeh, shoyu, sauerkraut, and other pickles are all good sources of *lactobacillus* bacteria. Miso and tempeh alone contain over 160 different bacteria strains. A plant-based diet, centered on whole grains and vegetables, will help prevent and relieve Crohn's, colitis, and other digestive ills.

CASE STUDIES

SARA'S STORY

I had been taking Asacol (Mesalamine) since I was 18 years old; gradually increasing the dosage to six pills, three times a day over the years as my condition worsened. Four years ago, since being on the macrobiotic diet, I went down to a low dose, two pills, three times a day because I was feeling so much better. One year ago, I went down to one pill, three times a day, this was against my doctors wishes. My doctor does encourage me to be on the macrobiotic diet, but he didn't want me off the medication. As of April this year, I have been completely off my medication. The last time I saw my doctor earlier this year; he said that I was doing so well on the diet that he did not need to see me again for another year. In sharing this discussion with my husband over dinner later that night, we both felt very confident in my progress so that motivated me to try going off my medication entirely.

My flare-ups are usually triggered by not getting ample sleep, eating without mindfulness, internalizing stressful situations, and overnight travel. Pre-flare symptoms typically include a little blood, mucus, bloating, diarrhea or constipation, and flatulence. I use my intuition and instinct, and check in with my macrobiotic counselor. I will make some adjustments in my diet and lifestyle. I will make the Ume-Sho-Kuzu drink, chew at least 50 times each mouthful and I am committed to chewing 150 times each mouthful at least one meal a day. Overall, I feel great and am happy to know the macrobiotic diet to guide me in managing my condition. I will be sharing my story at this year's Kushi Institute Summer Conference. I will be on the *Celebrating Life* panel and hope to see you there.

Source: KushiInstitute.org

VIRGINIA HARPER

"You can turn this around. You can change this," are the words I'll never forget. After eight years of living with Takayasu's arteritis and Crohn's disease and seeing only a dim future ahead, these words filled me with hope.

At age 14 I started having strong symptoms of discomfort and pain on the right side of my abdomen. At 15 they removed my appendix but discovered it was normal. From 15 to 23, I was in and out of hospitals at least twice a year with the symptoms getting more severe. I had not only the increasing abdominal problems but I started to develop fainting spells, dizziness, weakness in my right shoulder and arm down to my hand. At age 19 I discovered a lump on my neck. I was away at college in Tennessee and the school doctor decided it was a benign cyst and could be easily removed during the Thanksgiving holidays.

While undergoing an arteriogram at home in Connecticut, I suffered a stroke. When I awoke, I was temporarily paralyzed on my right side and had lost my ability to speak. The test showed a blockage on my right carotid artery. In April of that next year, I was sent to Mass General Hospital in Boston to undergo bypass surgery and a biopsy and it was determined that I had a very rare blood condition. Takayasu arteritis is an autoimmune deficiency where the blood passing through the arteries causes them to act as if they are damaged so they start repairing themselves and this creates blockages. Takayasu has no known cause and no known cure. The main arteries were so dramatically affected that my blood flow was distressed. I was told to stop all my sports activities and "to take it easy." But the real devastating news was that I should not plan on having children.

I was put on an anti-inflammatory drug called prednisone, a steroid, and an aspirin a day to help with my blood flow. The next few years I learned to live within the confines of Takayasu and I suffered from the side effects from the drug more than the disease itself. I would awaken ravished with headaches, swollen aching joints, ringing in my ears, upset stomach, low energy and feeling depressed. And, when I was on high doses, I would be so hyper I would work to exhaustion and still only need three or four hours of sleep before I was ready to go again.

On top of all this, my abdominal symptoms began to get worse as the years went by. The pain became paralyzing, along with constant headaches, bloody diarrhea, constipation and weight loss. At times I would lose so much blood that I would go to the emergency room completely debilitated. The X-rays showed nothing. Eight years of different doctors, specialists, tests, and drugs, yet the cause and cure were still a mystery.

Finally, when I was 22, I had a severe attack that landed me back in the emergency room. But this time, the technicians were finally able to detect something on the X-rays. The doctors diagnosed Crohn's disease. I was so relieved to have a name for what I had gone through all those years. Crohn's disease has no known cause and no known cure. It causes a slow deterioration of the intestinal wall, the lining become inflamed and irritated, and loses its elasticity resulting in impaired digestion and absorption. Crohn's can manifest anywhere in the digestive tract.

Anti-inflammatory drugs and/or surgery were the only recourse. Surgery can remove the affected area; however, Crohn's usually spreads again in three years or less and you will face more surgery. It didn't take me long to realize that if I lived to be 30, I would not have any intestines left.

The "good news" was that I was already taking the anti-inflammatory drug used to treat it. When I inquired how I could develop something so severe when I was already on the drug that supposedly helped it, I got no response. And so, I learned to live within the confines of Crohn's and Prednisone.

To complicate matters, that same year I became pregnant while using the IUD. Instead of this being a happy time for my husband and me, it was quite traumatic. The doctors thought I would lose the baby when they removed the IUD. However, the pregnancy continued and went smoothly while the doctors watched me very closely and I stayed in bed most of the time. Being as determined as I am, our beautiful daughter was born.

Nine months later, the Takayasu and the Crohn's both flared up again and so did my trips back to the hospital and doctors for more tests and different drugs, except this time nothing seemed to work for very long. My parents and I, being open to alternative methods, started searching for real cures. I tried megavitamin therapy, reflexology, herbs, and hospital-based nutritional approaches. It was during this search that my father heard about macrobiotics. He cried as he told me what would work this time and shared what little he knew. He flew me to Connecticut to see a macrobiotic teacher. I was ready to deal with this doctor, too. I took all my X-rays, files, and paperwork to show him, but the experience was totally different.

He wanted to know specific details of my symptoms and my lifestyle. There was no prodding, poking, sticking, undressing, or cold intrusive instruments to deal with. He used Oriental diagnosis to evaluate my condition by observing my eyes, tongue, hands, and feet. Finally, he told me what I had longed to hear, "You can turn this around."

The macrobiotic teacher proceeded to explain that there were certain foods that weakened my body and it was struggling to get rid of excess. All my body needed were the correct tools to naturally heal itself. The main foods that aggravated my condition were dairy food and sugars.

For maximum health, he explained the importance of keeping the body alkaline by eating neutral or balanced foods. These include whole grains, beans, land and sea vegetables, and some fruit, seeds, and nuts.

I grew up with my grandmother and she strongly believed that God's abundance provides everything one needs to naturally heal. All I heard finally was making sense. I did not recognize half of the foods he mentioned because after all, I was a fast food, junk food, and pre-prepared, vegetables-come-in-a-can, baby-boomer.

I had answers and most of all, for the first time, I had hope. My teacher told me that one-day I would appreciate and be thankful for my illness. I thought, "This guy has been eating too much seaweed he just doesn't realize all I've been through!"

Now, years later, I continue to live a symptom-free, drug-free, pain-free, doctor-free life. Full of energy, I anticipate a health-filled future with my two children and family. I truly understand those prophetic words. I do appreciate my illness and all I went through. My experience led me to macrobiotics and that led me to the path of healing physically, emotionally, and spiritually.

Source: KushiInistute.org

MARISA MARINELLI

Halfway through class I begin to struggle. I walk away from the ballet barre and sit down in the corner, no longer able to ignore the unease and discomfort in my stomach. My

Advanced Ballet III professor approaches me after class, concerned about my behavior. "This might sound weird," I say to him, "but I feel like I can't feel my stomach, like it's numb." With a look of skepticism and obvious condescendence he replies with minimal sensitivity. "Well, I just think you have a weak center."

That memory has always stuck with me; my professor, even with his hint of arrogance, was correct about my weak center. I was a 19-year-old college student, training to become a professional dancer, when I was diagnosed with an Inflammatory Bowel Disease. I wasn't aware of it at the time, but the numbness I had been feeling was the beginnings of severe inflammation of the colon.

I have actually been told I'm lucky. It only took two colonoscopies for my doctor to say, "Good news! You don't have Crohn's disease, it's only ulcerative colitis." If that's "luck," I wonder what winning the lottery is like. Having never heard of either disease, at that time I couldn't understand how my life would never be the same.

It's been a seven-year journey of struggles and success, but today I finally understand that my health was not a matter of "luck"- it was a matter of choice. I was fortunate enough to have learned about macrobiotics; to have the option to choose an alternative healing path, I chose to heal.

After my diagnosis I suffered immensely for several years. Flare-ups would come and go monthly and I'd find myself in the hospital for weeks at a time. Severe diarrhea and vomiting caused me to loose so much weight and muscle mass. I had difficulty walking, let alone dancing. I never knew what to eat and I was always in pain. My doctors would treat me with powerful, harsh anti-inflammatory drugs to ease my bouts of illness.

I wouldn't offer a dose of prednisone to even my worst enemy. The side effects are torturous. I sacrificed whatever healthy organs I had left to prednisone.

One year after my diagnosis I learned, in addition to the ulcerative colitis, I was one the 5% of all IBD patients in the world to develop a secondary reaction to the disease called Pyoderma Gangrenosum. In this rare instance, inflammation is no longer contained in the colon; it is systemic.

Ulcers can begin to develop on my limbs. If ulceration grows into the bones, the doctors would have no choice but to amputate that limb. Being that my case was so rare, my doctor had never treated or met a patient with these conditions. Confused, he believed that I was the worst case of ulcerative colitis he had ever seen.

Extreme high dosages of prednisone seemed to be necessary to put me into a temporary remission. Because I had a strong, dancer's body, I survived the first huge flare with all my limbs and no surgery. However, a few months after I was off the drug, I would relapse into the same cycle and find myself back in the hospital.

I feared that this drug-dependent life was the only choice I had.
Surgery was never an option for me. Call me superficial, but I wasn't willing to part with any of my body parts.

Drugs were not the answer; they would only weaken my immune system and that's not something I'm willing to sacrifice. And, who wants to take 20 pills a day for the rest of their life? Doctors could not offer me any other hope, so I began to look for alternative options. Macrobiotics was my answer.

I became friends with a young girl, who also suffered with ulcerative colitis. She gave me a book to read called *Controlling Crohn's Disease The Natural Way*. The book is written by Virginia Harper, a woman who healed her Crohn's disease through a macrobiotic-based diet and lifestyle. I read the book, cover to cover, in 2 days. "This makes sense," I thought. "I have nothing left to loose, so I might as well give it a try."

I never imagined my body being "off balance." Can sea vegetables and brown rice really make a difference to my body? I found Virginia's website and contacted her for a consultation as soon as possible. Macrobiotics provided a new hope for me, and a new life.

Hope is great, but I needed more hands-on guidance.
Although Virginia Harper became my "guru" of digestive diseases, she was located geographically too far for me to travel at that time. I decided to go to the source of macrobiotics, the Kushi Institute in Becket, MA. You're talking to a girl who didn't even know how to boil rice, let along know what the word "blanching" meant. I needed some drastic help on my understanding of cooking and philosophy. I signed up for the Way To Health Program

in February 2006. There's no understatement here, this program completely changed my life. After 10 days of living in the Berkshires, I returned to NYC a different person, AND my symptoms were going away! I learned about a plant-based diet, yin and yang theory, how to cut vegetables, and most important, WHY any of this information is important to our health and well-being. With the information I was given from Kushi Institute's program, I had the motivation to set myself on a strict "healing program" for myself. It's more than just dietary changes that need to take place. I needed to learn that if I was patient with myself, every day, in every way, I will get better and better.

Nobody says change is easy.
Being from a first-generation Italian family, food is a huge part of our culture. We love it and can't get enough of it. Pasta, cheese, and tomato sauce were my main food groups. If you didn't lick your plate clean, Nonna (or "grand-mother," in Italian) would chase you around the kitchen with that last bite on her spoon.

I never thought about how food affected my body because I was always very thin and fit. When I told my family I was changing my diet drastically, they had no idea how big of change I intended.

With family and friends, I suddenly became the "weird girl" who didn't eat meat or dairy. I'll never forget the time I went to the beach and a friend jokingly asked if "I was going to eat the seaweed for lunch?"

For someone who didn't want to change her diet in the first place, it was very difficult to find motivation to keep on this path. Not only were the comments, and sometimes jokes, hurtful; I didn't know how to cook! The first time I had to make brown rice I asked my mom, "How does it cook?" I couldn't pronounce any of the foreign foods, or find them at my local supermarket. An ume-what plum? But the biggest boost of confidence and motivation was that IT WORKED!

Within the first month of committing to whole grain, beans and vegetables, my symptoms were gone and I was jumping out of bed in the morning. After a few more months on a macrobiotic approach, I saw a huge difference in myself; more energy, calmer moods, better sleep and I was happy! I was able to return to dance and enjoy it more than ever.

My story doesn't end there.

Making the change to a macrobiotic diet and lifestyle was, and still is, one of the hardest things I've done in my life. Even after seven years there are continuous ups and downs. Thankfully, however, it gets easier. The great new is, I have the rest of my life ahead of me to live fully. There was a time of my life where I thought life wasn't worth living if you couldn't enjoy some macaroni and cheese; I was wrong. Honestly, today, I can say I don't miss it.

The rewards of eating good food push me through the hardest of times. Don't forget your support group. People come into (and leave) your life for a reason. I have learned to take every experience for what it is, and then let go. Stay close to those that are truly supportive. Family is forever, but it's okay to disagree when it comes to what's best for you.

It's during the most challenging parts of life that a person needs to be the strongest and make the wisest, and often most difficult, of choices. I chose to be thankful for my disease. I wanted to heal myself: mind, body and soul. I made the decision to do whatever it took to find a way to heal myself because I was NOT going to spend any more of my life being ill. I was, and still am, a young adult with lots of ambition and dreams. My body was weak; my will power was not.

I've witness many people; faced with a serious health issue, turn away from hope. "This isn't an option for me" or "It's too hard." We all have a choice in our life to create our own destiny and it's up to us to decide what we want that to be.

I've made the choice to heal and hope to inspire others to do the same. I've chosen food and life over doctors, drugs and surgeries. I've learned at a young age that if you don't have your health, you really don't have anything at all.

To those who are lucky enough to come across my story, please know for life and health, you always have a choice.

Source: MacroMarinelli.com

MICHELLE DAVIS-LEVY

My name is Michelle Davis-Levy. I came to the Kushi Institute back in 2014 after 16 years of dealing with Crohn's disease. I had just had my ileum (lower small intestine) removed and my two year-old son had become my caretaker because Crohn's disease was that debilitating. I went to work every day wearing pull-ups to make sure that I didn't soil myself on the train. I was not able to eat anything that sustained my body. I was very skinny and very unhealthy and always very sad because I was told that Crohn's was incurable; I would never be able to eat anything that I really enjoyed and I would never be able to enjoy my children and my family because I was always weak. My life revolved around the toilet!

I attended the *Controlling Crohn's and Colitis* seminar with Virginia Harper and it changed my life. Virginia gave me not just practical tools but tools that resounded with me, it helped me with my faith, things that let me know that not only am I going to have a good life, but also I will be able to do things that tell me that doctors don't know everything. I am a divine soul and my body is meant not only to heal but also to regenerate itself.

I learned how to eat things that give me strength and strengthen my body, and that give me the opportunity to lead a normal life with my now five year-old son. I recently taught him how to ride his bike. I can go running with him and not be exhausted after five minutes. I drove here without having to plot out where the bathrooms were. That's freedom when you are a Crohn's patient. And it's a freedom I don't take for granted.

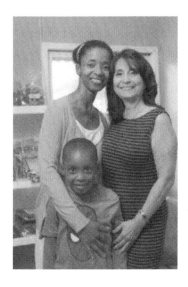

Michelle Davis-Levy (left) with Virginia Harper.
Photo: Nancy Adler

As of August 2016 I will be starting my Masters Degree in Social Work program. I didn't think I'd be able to do that because stress in a Crohn's patient's life creates bodily harm and for me school was always stressful. Now I have things that show me what my triggers are, teach me how to heal my gut so that when I go through school I am going to school empowered. I can balance my energy. I know what to do to take care of myself and so I am no longer a patient with Crohn's disease who spends majority of her time at the doctors and taking pills. Now I am a healthy and vibrant woman pursuing her education while leading a happy and healthy life.

Source: Kushi Institute Newsletter

CASSIE'S STORY

Paula Pini

Cassie M. (names have been changed to protect the privacy of the individuals involved) joined our library staff in the winter of 2017. She had been working with us at our small community college in the Northeast for a few months when one summer day I received an email from Cassie explaining that she would be out of work for a while, due to the fact that she was hospitalized and it was suspected that she had Crohn's disease. Within six months of her return to work, I started my macrobiotic studies with Edward Esko, director of the International Macrobiotic Institute, and was happy to share what I was learning with Cassie in hopes of helping her. I learned more about Cassie and her battle with Crohn's, and I discovered that she had a family history of the disease. This is Cassie's story.

During the 1970s and 1980s Cassie watched her father, John, deal with a very serious condition known as Crohn's disease. He had been diagnosed with this disease while he was in high school and had been having Crohn's symptoms for years. Crohn's disease is an inflammatory bowel disease (IBD) that can manifest anywhere in the gastrointestinal tract, but most commonly affects the terminal ileum, the connecting point between the small and the large intestine on the right side of the colon. People suffering from the disease can experience abdominal pain, cramping, diarrhea, bloody stools, fevers, and a feeling of fatigue. In macrobiotics, Crohn's disease is classified as having more yin characteristics, with the major causes being chicken, cheese and milk.

Prior to Cassie's father being diagnosed with the disease, he drank a lot of milk. Cassie thinks he was drinking a lot of milk because he also suffered with ulcers. John eventually gave up milk, but continued eating chicken and cheese. Over time, Cassie watched her father go through multiple surgeries, some of them emergency surgeries, where portions of his intestine were removed in hopes of healing his condition. John had to swallow "handfuls of pills" every day, with Prednisone, a steroid drug that treats a number of conditions where inflammation is present, being the only drug that could control Crohn's disease. In addition to the Crohn's, John also developed osteoporosis. In 2004, ten days after that last surgery, John died in intensive care. He was 58 years old. John ultimately passed from complications resulting from the surgery, and, Cassie believes, complications resulting from his many treatments and medications.

In 2016 Cassie started to get headaches. She considered herself a fairly healthy person and would take probiotics, on and off. Antibiotics were prescribed for a skin condition, but otherwise she never had any major illnesses or medical problems. But the headaches persisted so she started taking Advil. She was feeling lethargic too, and had no energy for running, an activity she enjoyed. Cassie ate dairy products and drank a lot of milk while she was pregnant, and ate cheese. Lots of cheese. She also ate meat, mostly chicken, for dinners and from the deli, to be eaten in sandwiches. She did eat vegetables.

When she started her new part-time job at the community college she was still not feeling well and she started having cramping and abdominal pain but no bowel symptoms. Her doctor suspected a urinary tract infection (UTI) and prescribed antibiotics, but the antibiotics did not work. The cramping and abdominal pain persisted. Her doctor recommended she go to the emergency room where a CT-scan was ordered. The imaging showed an intra-abdominal abscess (IAA). This is an infection within the abdomen that can be caused by a number of conditions such as appendicitis, a bowel rupture, Crohn's or ulcerative colitis. Surgery and trauma could also be a cause. The UTI the doctor thought Cassie had was bacteria from the IAA.

At the time the ER doctors thought she might have a ruptured appendix and she was admitted to the hospital where she was started on IV fluids and antibiotics. At one point the surgeons discussed draining the abscess but they didn't, to Cassie's relief. Cassie was in the hospital for three days where it was determined that a ruptured appendix did not cause the infection. She was given more antibiotics and referred to a GI doctor. At this point there was no absolute diagnosis of Crohn's but it was suspected. After she was discharged she had a follow-up visit with the GI doctor and repeat imaging showed no signs of the abscess. Blood work was ordered and genetic markers for Crohn's disease were confirmed. A colonoscopy followed and the results showed a deep abdominal ulcer. The results of a biopsy were consistent with Crohn's disease.

The first thing the doctors wanted to do was put Cassie on Humira. Humira is an immunosuppressive drug that is prescribed for a number of conditions, including Crohn's. (Global sales of Humira topped 19.9 billion in 2018 according to AbbVie, the company that produces the drug.) Before Cassie agrees to take this drug she does her own research on it, and other drugs that are given to treat this disease. She tells her GI doctor that she wants to try Entocort, another steroid drug instead because it is formulated to release in the gut, which limits the systemic effects. With other steroids, the drug effects other parts of the body. Her doctor reacts favorably to Cassie's suggestion and she takes it from fall to Christmas of 2016.

When Cassie was hospitalized I had already started my macrobiotic studies. I was learning how dairy, meats, and sugar affect the human body both physically and energetically. When I learned that she had been diagnosed with Crohn's disease I asked her what she was eating. I even showed her my class notes and a diagram that showed where in the colon that Crohn's normally manifests. My scribbled notes on the paper read: "chicken, milk, cheese." "That's it" Cassie said when she saw my class notes, "That's exactly what I was eating!" When we eat conventional factory farmed meat and dairy foods, I explained, we are taking into our bodies the suffering and sadness of their lives. We are also taking in the antibiotics that are given to the animals to prevent illness.

Cassie eliminates all dairy, all meat, and all caffeine. I encourage her to add more brown rice, miso soups, and vegetables in her diet. I think this gave her a bit of added courage to trust her own instincts about her body. Now, Cassie eats lots of vegetables, stir fries, brown rice, pasta and beans such as chickpeas. She takes probiotics and adds miso to soups. She also eliminates Advil, which she had been taking on a regular basis to help with her headaches. Because a common side effect of Advil is gastrointestinal upset and ulcers, Cassie vows to "never take it again."

As Cassie's health improves, the Entocort steroid is gradually tapered off. Her doctor wants her to take a maintenance medicine to keep the Crohn's from flaring up, and Cassie suggests Pentasa. Already familiar with the nonsteroidal anti-inflammatory drug, she discovers that her health insurance company will not cover the costs. Cassie appeals this decision but the health insurance company will still not cover it. Cassie then decides that she doesn't want any other drugs. She tells her doctor: "I'm okay with not being on anything." Cassie was not expecting her doctor's reaction to her decision. She looked at Cassie like she was a child, or incredibly dense, and said "You have a chronic disease." Cassie was not deterred. She was trusting her instincts, eating better and taking probiotics. She had seen what the conventional medical protocol for treating Crohn's disease had done to her father. No dietary advice was ever given to her. When Cassie asked about what she should eat, her doctor shrugged. "Avoid spicy food, fried food." That was it.

Today, Cassie eats lots of vegetables, the prebiotics that feed the probiotics, and listens to stress relieving music. She is an avid churchgoer, and prayer is important to her. She takes no medicine for Crohn's disease and is happy, healthy and disease free. She remembers the day she was released from the hospital, Monday, August 21, 2017. It was a very special day as the earth was experiencing a total solar eclipse of the sun. "It was surreal," Cassie says. A group of doctors were standing together looking at the eclipse through special filtered glasses. The symbolism was perfect.

Macrobiotics

Standard Dietary and Way of Life
Suggestions
For persons living in a temperate climate

Daily Dietary Recommendations
WHOLE CEREAL GRAINS. At least 50% by weight of every meal is recommended to include cooked, organically grown, whole cereal grains prepared in a variety of ways. Whole cereal grains include brown rice, barley, millet, whole wheat, rye, oats, corn, and buckwheat. Please note that a portion of this amount may consist of noodles or pasta, unyeasted whole grain breads, and other partially processed whole cereal grains.

SOUPS. Approximately 5-10% of your daily food intake may include soup made with vegetables, sea vegetables (wakame or kombu) grains, or beans. Seasonings are usually miso or shoyu (organic soy sauce.) The flavor should not be too salty.

VEGETABLES. About 25-30% of daily intake may include local and organically grown vegetables. Preferably, the majority is cooked in various styles (e.g. sautéed with a small amount of vegetable oil, steamed, boiled, and sometimes as raw salad or naturally fermented or pickled vegetables.

Vegetables for daily use include green cabbage, kale, broccoli, cauliflower, collards, pumpkin, watercress, Chinese cabbage, bok choy, dandelion, mustard greens, daikon greens, scallion, onion, daikon, turnip, various fall and summer squashes, burdock, carrot, varieties.

Avoid or limit the intake of potato (including sweet potato and yam), tomato, eggplant, pepper, spinach, asparagus, beet, zucchini, and avocado. Mayonnaise and other oily, fatty, or artificial dressings are best avoided.

BEANS AND SEA VEGETABLES. Approximately 5-10% of the daily diet may include cooked beans and sea vegetables. Beans for regular use include azuki, chickpea, lentil, and black soybean, as well as kidney, navy, black bean, white beans, pinto, non-GMO soybean, and others. Bean products such as tofu, tempeh, and natto can also be used. Sea vegetables such as wakame, nori, kombu, hiziki, arame, dulse, agar, and others may be prepared in a variety of ways. They can be cooked with beans or vegetables, used in soups, or served separately as side dishes or salads, moderately flavored with brown rice vinegar, sea salt, shoyu, ume plum, and other natural seasonings.

OCCASIONAL FOODS. If needed or desired, 1-3 times a week, approximately 10% of the daily consumption of food can include fresh wild caught flaky white meat fish. Non-farm raised salmon and sea scallops can be included several times per month if your condition permits.

Fruit or fruit desserts, including fresh, dried, and cooked fruits, may also be served three or four times per week on average. Local and organically grown fruits are preferred. If you live in a temperate climate, avoid tropical and semi-tropical fruit and eat, instead, temperate climate fruits such as apples, pears, plums, peaches, nectarines, apricots, berries, and melons. Local organic fruit juice may also be consumed if your condition permits.

Lightly roasted nuts and seeds such as pumpkin, sesame, and sunflower may be enjoyed as snacks, together with peanuts, walnuts, almonds, and pecans.

Rice syrup, barley malt, amasake, and mirin may be used as sweeteners, together with occasional maple syrup. Brown rice vinegar, lemon, or umeboshi vinegar may be used for a sour taste.

BEVERAGES. Recommended daily beverages include bancha (kukicha) twig tea, stem tea, roasted brown rice and barley tea, and occasional dandelion and corn silk tea. Any traditional tea that does not have an aromatic fragrance or a stimulating effect can be used. You may also drink a comfortable amount of water (preferably spring or well water of good quality) but not iced.

FOODS TO REDUCE OR AVOID. Meat, animal fat, eggs, poultry, dairy products (including butter, yogurt, ice cream, milk, and cheese), refined sugars, chocolate, molasses, honey, other simple sugars like stevia, agave, evaporated cane juice, etc., and foods treated with them.

Tropical or semi-tropical fruits and fruit juices, including banana and pineapple, soda, artificial drinks and beverages, coffee, colored tea, and all aromatic stimulating teas such as mint or peppermint.

All artificially colored, preserved, sprayed, or chemically treated foods, including foods with GMO ingredients. All refined and polished grains, flours, and their derivatives. Mass-produced industrialized food including canned, frozen, and irradiated foods.

Hot spices, any aromatic stimulating food or food accessory, artificial vinegar, and strong alcoholic beverages, especially those produced from sugar or mixed with sugared beverages.

ADDITIONAL SUGGESTIONS. Cooking oil should be vegetable quality only, with natural cold pressed olive and sesame as preferred varieties.

Salt should be naturally processed sea salt. Traditional, non-chemical shoyu or tamari soy sauce and miso may be used as seasonings.

Recommended condiments include:

—Gomashio (sesame salt made from approx. 20 parts roasted sesame seeds to one part sea salt)

—Sea vegetable powder or flakes, including green

nori, dulse, kelp, wakame and others, as well as combinations or blends.

   —Sesame seed wakame powder

   —Umeboshi plum

   —Tekka

   —Roasted seeds such as sunflower or pumpkin

Pickled vegetables made without sugar or strong spice, including non-pasteurized organic sauerkraut, pickled Chinese cabbage, and others may be eaten on a daily basis.

You may have meals regularly, 2-3 times per day, as much as you want, provided the proportion is correct and the chewing is thorough. Avoid eating for approximately 3 hours before sleeping.

THE IMPORTANCE OF COOKING. Proper cooking is very important for health. Everyone should learn to cook either by attending classes or under the guidance of an experienced macrobiotic cook. The recipes included in macrobiotic cookbooks may also be used in planning meals.

SPECIAL ADVICE

The guidelines present above are general suggestions. These suggestions may require modification depending on your individual condition. Of course, any serious condition should be closely monitored by the appropriate medical, nutritional, and health professional.

Together with beginning to change your diet, we invite you to attend regular seminars, cooking classes, and study programs and to meet with a qualified macrobiotic counselor or educator.

Way of Life Suggestions

- Live each day happily without being preoccupied with your health; try to keep mentally and physically active.
- View everything and everyone you meet with gratitude, particularly offering thanks before and after each meal.
- Chew your food very well, at least 50 times per mouthful, or until it becomes liquid.
- It is best to retire before midnight and get up early every morning.
- It is best to avoid wearing synthetic or woolen clothing directly on the skin. As much as possible, wear cotton, especially for undergarments. Avoid excessive metallic accessories on the fingers, wrists, or neck. Keep such ornaments simple and graceful.
- Take a ½ hour walk each day. When safe and appropriate, walk barefoot on grass, beach, or soil. Keep your home in good order, from the kitchen, bathroom, bedroom, and living quarters, to every corner of the house.
- Initiate and maintain an active correspondence, extending your best wishes to parents, children, brothers and sisters, teachers, and friends.

- Avoid taking long hot showers or baths unless you have been consuming too much salt or animal food.
- To increase circulation, scrub your entire body with a hot, damp towel very morning or every night. If that is not possible, at least scrub your hands, feet, fingers and toes.
- Avoid chemically perfumed cosmetics. For care of the teeth, brush with natural, fluoride-free preparations.
- If your condition permits, exercise regularly as part of daily life, including activities like walking, scrubbing floors, cleaning windows, washing clothes and working in the garden. You may also participate in exercise programs such as yoga, martial arts, dance, or sports.
- Avoid using electric cooking devices (stoves, ovens, ranges) or microwave ovens. Convert to gas cooking at the earliest opportunity.
- It is best to minimize the use of color television, computer monitors, cellphones, tablets, smartphones, and other mobile devices.
- Include large green plants in your house to freshen and enrich the oxygen content of the air in your home. Open windows frequently to permit air to circulate freely.
- Sing a happy song every day.

SPECIAL DISHES AND REMEDIES

Specific for Crohn's and Colitis

The recipes in this section have special benefits for persons with Crohn's and colitis. They represent only a small sample of the hundreds and even thousands of dishes that are available in the macrobiotic diet. These dishes and remedies are not a complete meal plan but represent featured dishes in a broad-based and varied macrobiotic way of eating. Please consult the books in the Recommended Reading section for a more complete diet plan. Contact the International Macrobiotic Institute for more information.

BROWN RICE
Basic brown rice can be the staple grain for daily use. It has tonifying and strengthening effects on the digestive system, and especially the colon (large intestine.) Whole, unrefined grains like millet, barley, whole wheat, and others can be used as supplements to daily brown rice.

1. Wash 1 cup of organic brown rice by covering with water, rinsing, and draining the water. Repeat three times.

2. Place in a pot with a tight-fitting lid.
3. Add a small pinch of sea salt and one and one-half to two cups of spring water (filtered water may also be used.)
4. Cover and bring to a boil on a medium high flame.
5. When the rice comes to an active boil, reduce the flame to low and cook for 50-60 minutes.
6. Turn off the flame and let the rice sit for several minutes.
7. Remove from the pot with a wooden spoon and place in a serving bowl.

Brown rice may be cooked in a pressure cooker. Bring 1 cup of washed grain to a boil in 1 1/2 cups water and when pressure is up, place a flame deflector under the pot. Lower the flame and cook for 50 minutes. Brown rice and other whole grains can also be soaked prior to cooking.

SOFT RICE KAYU

You may make soft rice porridge (kayu) from leftover cooked grain by adding 2-3 times the amount of water and boiling it gently (covered with a lid) until it softens and becomes a porridge-like consistency. You may eat porridge with crumbled toasted nori, dulse or other seaweed flakes or powder, umeboshi plum or paste, gomashio or other suggested condiments. Garnish with fresh chopped scallion, parsley, or chive. Organic brown rice syrup or other natural sweeteners can be used to sweeten rice, oat, or other organic whole grain breakfast porridges on occasion. You may complement your breakfast with a variety of quickly boiled vegetables (Chinese cabbage, leafy greens, etc.) and miso soup if you wish.

BASIC MISO SOUP
Use high-quality miso, fermented over at least two summers, as your primary staple. For everyday use, barley miso (mugi miso) is best. For variation, you may use soybean miso (hatcho miso) or brown rice miso (genmai miso). Specialty handcrafted miso such as chickpea, dandelion-leek, azuki bean, and others may be used from time to time, as well as red, yellow, white, or other shorter-fermented miso, provided their ingredients are natural and organic.

1. Soak wakame (one-quarter to one-half inch piece per person) for about five minutes and cut into small pieces.
2. Soak dried shiitake mushroom (one mushroom per cup of liquid) for about five minutes and cut into small pieces, removing the hard stem.
3. Add the wakame and shiitake to fresh, cold water and bring to a boil. Meanwhile, cut some vegetables into small pieces. Add to the wakame and shiitake stock. Recommendations include: daikon, carrot and onion, kabocha (or other sweet squash), other fresh, local, and organic vegetables such as those listed in the previous section.
4. Add the vegetables to the boiling broth and boil all

together for three to five minutes until the vegetables are soft and edible. Reduce flame to low.

5. Dilute miso (one-half to one level teaspoon per cup of broth) in a little water, add to soup, and simmer for three to four minutes on a low flame. The broth should not have a harsh salty taste. Please note that it is important not to bring the soup to a boil once the miso has been added.

6. Garnish each bowl or serving with fresh chopped scallion, chive, or parsley.

DRIED DAIKON WITH CARROT AND ONION

Daikon aids in the discharge of fat and liquid, thus aiding in strengthening and cleansing the colon. Carrot, daikon, and other root vegetables are used to strengthen and heal the colon. The naturally sweet flavor of this dish reduces the desire for refined sugar and artificial sweets.

1. Soak 1/2 cup of dried daikon for about 10 minutes or until it is soft. If the dried daikon has a very dark color and the water is also dark, discard the water. If the water is a light color, you may use it in the dish.

2. Place the dried daikon (chopped if desired) in the pot and add enough water to cover.

3. Cut equal amounts of carrot and onion into thin slices. The amount of vegetables can equal the amount of daikon.

4. Cover the pot, bring to a boil, and lower the flame.

Simmer for 20-30 minutes until the vegetables are tender.

5. Season lightly with shoyu (organic soy sauce) and cook until excess liquid evaporates.

AZUKI BEANS WITH SQUASH AND KOMBU

Azuki beans and kombu sea vegetable provide a slow steady release of glucose. They have been used for centuries to strengthen and vitalize the kidneys. Sweet fall or winter squash blends perfectly with the beans and sea vegetable. This dish strengthens the pancreas while easing the craving for sweets, and also aids in the formation of smooth, firm bowel movements.

1. Wash and soak ½ cup of azuki beans with a 1-inch piece of kombu sea vegetable (optional) for several hours or overnight.

2. Place the kombu in the bottom of a pot and add chopped hard winter or autumn squash, especially kabocha squash.

3. Add azuki beans to the pot.

4. Bring slowly to a boil without covering the pot. Cover after 10 to 15 minutes.

5. Cook on a low flame until the beans become soft, about an hour or more. The water evaporates as the beans expand, so add water from time to time to keep the level constant.

6. Add a few pinches of sea salt or shoyu to taste.

7. Cover and cook for 15 to 30 minutes or until most of the water has evaporated.

8. Turn off the flame and let sit for several minutes before serving. Garnish with finely chopped scallion.

STEAMED GREENS

(Kale, collards, watercress, mustard green, daikon green, turnip green, dandelion green, carrot tops, Chinese cabbage, bok choy, etc.)

1. Wash and slice any of the above vegetables.
2. Place vegetables in small amount of boiling water (one-half inch) or in a stainless steel steamer above about one inch of boiling water.
3. Cover and steam or boil for two to three minutes, depending on the texture of the vegetables.
4. Transfer quickly to a serving dish to prevent overcooking.

Notes:

The vegetables should be a bright green color and crispy.

Wait until the water is fully boiling before you put in the vegetables.

You may lightly sprinkle lemon or brown rice vinegar over the greens at the end.

When boiling, do not cover the pot with a lid or the greens will lose their bright green color.

SAUERKRAUT

Sauerkraut (fermented cabbage) and other pickled vegetable foods, including miso and natto (whole fermented soybeans) contain living bacteria and enzymes that strengthen the colonies of beneficial bacteria in the large intestine. They help to rebuild colon health. Look for organic unpasteurized varieties rich in probiotics. Companies such as Real Pickles, Bubbies, and Hosta Hill now offer organic unpasteurized lacto-fermented sauerkraut and pickles.

SESAME WAKAME CONDIMENT
Sea vegetables contain minerals that help alkalize the blood and strengthen the absorption of nutrients. Sea vegetables help contract and strengthen the intestines.

1. Roast wakame sea vegetable in a dry skillet over a medium flame until dark and crisp.
2. Grind into a fine powder in a clay-grinding bowl known as a suribachi.
3. Roast an equal amount of washed and rinsed sesame seeds in the dry skillet over medium heat. Use a wooden spoon to gently stir the seeds to avoid burning. The seeds will begin to pop when ready and give off a nutty fragrance. Lower the flame toward the end of cooking.
4. Add the seeds while hot to the suribachi with the crushed wakame. Slowly and gently grind with the wooden pestle until each seed is thoroughly crushed.
5. Store in an airtight container and sprinkle on brown rice and other grain dishes.

PREPARED SEAWEED CONDIMENTS

Maine Coast Sea Vegetable Company offers a variety of prepared sea vegetable condiments, all of which add valuable minerals and iodine to the diet while having low sodium content. They include Dulse, Kelp, and Triple Blend Sea Vegetable Flakes. They can be used daily on whole grain and other dishes.

UME-SHO-KUZU

Kuzu is a root starch thickener (see photo below) with strengthening properties. Umeboshi is a pickled plum with strong antibacterial, digestive strengthening, and alkalizing effects. Ume-Sho-Kuzu is a standard macrobiotic drink to strengthen digestion, restore energy, reduce inflammation, and help the body discharge acidity. It has a strong salty-sour taste.

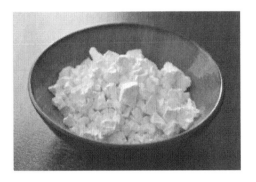

1. Dissolve 1 heaping teaspoon of kuzu in 2 to 3 teaspoons of cold water.
2. Add 1 cup of cold water to the dissolved kuzu.
3. Bring to a boil over a medium flame, stirring

constantly to prevent lumping, until the liquid becomes translucent. Reduce the flame to low.
4. Add the pulp of ½ to 1 umeboshi plum.
5. Add several drops to 1 teaspoon of shoyu and stir gently.
6. Simmer 2-3 minutes and drink hot.

SALT PACK

The Roasted Salt Pack is a gentle yet effective remedy for pain relief. Use it to heat and ease tension in various parts of the body (stiff muscles, the abdominal area in case of diarrhea, menstrual or intestinal cramps, stomach cramps, etc.)

1. Dry roast one to one and one-half cups of sea salt in a stainless steel skillet until it becomes hot. Test with your fingers from time to time to make sure it doesn't become too hot.
2. Pour the hot salt in a small or medium cotton towel and tie securely with a rubber band, string, or shoelace.
3. Apply to the affected area. Leave on until the salt cools.

You can reheat for subsequent applications. Save the salt as it can be used again. Eventually discard when the salt becomes gray and no longer holds heat, usually after four or five applications. You can use less expensive sea salt, such as that available at natural food stores and supermarkets, to prepare the salt pack.

HEALING DISHES

Virginia Harper

The Roasted Salt Pack and Ume-Sho-Kuzu are remedies previously mentioned that work immediately to help soothe active symptoms. The following recipes help in the gentle feeding and absorbing of concentrated nutrients. Due to the balanced nature of these dishes, they create energetic support for the digestive processes. Each dish has a nutritional and energetic benefit in absorption and digestion. They may be used as often as necessary and complement as side dishes any menu.

CREAMED RICE
Soothes and nourishes the activity of the intestines. This recipe is used for debilitating illness when digestion is impaired. In Asian and Latin cultures, soft cooked rice is used to soothe the belly.

Ingredients

> Short grain brown rice
> Spring water
> Kombu (hydrated)
> Umeboshi plum

Directions

Wash 1 cup of rice, then roast in a dry skillet, stirring until golden brown. Add 5 cups of spring water and a 2-inch piece of kombu. Bring to a boil, cover, and simmer on a low flame for 2 hours. Mill through a food mill or a strainer to extract into a fine cream. Serve with ½ to 1 full umeboshi plum chopped into the mixture.

NISHIME

Nishime is root vegetables chopped into small chunks and cooked until soft in their juices. This cooking method is strengthening for the blood and provides intestinal fortitude.

Ingredients

> Kombu (hydrated)
> Spring water
> Choice of vegetables: see suggestion list below
> Sea salt
> Shoyu

Directions

Use a heavy pot with a lid. Soak a 1/2- to 1-inch piece of kombu until soft and cut into 1/2-inch pieces. Place kombu in bottom of pot and cover with spring water. Add vegetables (see suggested combinations below.) The vegetables should be cut into 2-inch chunks except burdock and lotus root, which should be cut smaller.

Sprinkle a pinch of sea salt or shoyu over the vegetables. Cover and place on a high flame until there is a strong steam. Lower flame and cook peacefully for 20 to 30 minutes.

If water evaporates during cooking, add more water to the bottom of the pot. When each vegetable has become soft and fully cooked, add a few drops of shoyu and mix the vegetables. Replace cover and cook over a low flame for 2 to 5 minutes. Remove cover and turn off flame. Allow the vegetables sit for about 2 minutes. Try the following combinations:

Combinations of Vegetables

Kombu and onion
Onion, cabbage, carrot, squash (winter)
Leek, carrot
Daikon or turnip, parsnip
Daikon, lotus root
Carrot, cabbage, burdock
Daikon or turnip, shiitake mushroom

KINPIRA
Kinpira is very strengthening to the digestive tract. Prepared using two main vegetables this dish is tasty and easily digested.

Ingredients

Sesame oil
Carrot
Burdock

Spring water
Shoyu or Tamari

Directions
Prepare into thinly cut matchstick pieces equal parts of burdock and carrots. Lightly brush sesame oil in a skillet (preferably cast iron). Bring to heat in a medium flame and add burdock. Cook burdock 2-3 minutes and then layer the carrots on top of the burdock. Lightly cover the bottom of the skillet with spring water, just enough to cover the burdock. Cover and cook until the vegetables reach desired softness, minimum 20 minutes. Once ready, turn off flame and add a small amount of shoyu or tamari for a light taste. Stir and cover until ready to eat.

KANTEN
Kanten is a delicious and light vegan jelled dessert. Made with agar-agar, a sea vegetable processed into flakes or a powder. Its medicinal benefit is to relax the intestines and support normal easy bowel movements.

Ingredients

Apple juice
Spring water
Agar flakes
Kuzu

Directions
In a small pot simmer 2/3 cup of apple juice, 1/3 cup of

water and 1 tablespoon of agar flakes until the agar has dissolved. Dissolve 1 level teaspoon of kuzu in a few tablespoons of water and stir into heated mixture and stir until it thickens and the kuzu turns transparent. Place in a dish and allow to gel. Refrigeration is not necessary, as it will gel at room temperature.

Resources

Berkshire Holistic Associates, Berkshire Holistic Associates (BHA) is a division of the non-profit Planetary Health, Inc, a Berkshire-based 501(c)(3) educational organization. Founded by Edward Esko, Alex Jack, and Bettina Zumdick, BHA is dedicated to providing quality and affordable education on the benefits of a plant-based way of eating. BHA also supports adoption of complementary approaches such as acupuncture, massage, Asian bodywork, and yoga, and serves as a referral for these services in Berkshire County. BHA is working with Berkshire Health Systems, a leading healthcare provider in western Mass., to develop a plant-based intervention study for Type 2 diabetes. Visit: www.BerkshireHolistic.com.

Planetary Health/Amberwaves, PO Box 487, Becket MA 01223, 413-623- 0012, email: shenwa@bcn.net, www.amberwaves.org. A grassroots network devoted to preserving amber waves of grain and keeping America and the planet beautiful through macrobiotic education and research. PH is a 501(c)(3) non-profit organization. It publishes books and articles by macrobiotic authors, educators, and Planetary Health co-founders, Alex Jack and Edward Esko, and sponsors the annual Macrobiotic

Summer Conference and research on the macrobiotic way of life.

International Macrobiotic Institute, MacrobioticOnlineCourse. com, InternationalMacrobioticInstitute.com. Worldwide macrobiotic education. Headquartered in Massachusetts, with affiliates in New York, Dubai, Abu Dhabi, Barcelona, Vietnam, Australia, and Kuala Lumpur. Seminars and online study programs with Edward Esko and associates.

Macrobiotics Today/George Ohsawa Macrobiotic Foundation (GOMF), 1277 Marian Ave., Chico CA 95928, 800-232-2372, www.OhsawaMacrobiotics.com. A macrobiotic publisher and educational center on the West Coast.

Virginia M. Harper
You Can Heal You...one meal at a time, Franklin, Tennessee. 615-646-2841. Personalized counseling and residential program focused on inflammatory bowel disease and autoimmune disorders. www.youcanhealyou.com

Barnard Medical Center
5100 Wisconsin Ave. N.W., Suite #401
Washington, D.C. 20016
202-527-7500
202-527-7400 (fax)

The Barnard Medical Center combines medical care with the latest advances in prevention and nutrition to create a health care plan designed for each client. If you need to treat and reverse diabetes, heart disease, high blood pressure, or other chronic conditions, the Barnard Medical Center will help you revolutionize your health.

Sommer White, M.D.
Vitality Medical Center, 125 Belle Forest Circle, Suite 100, Nashville, TN 37221. Tel: 615-891-7500, www.sommer-whitemd.com. Holistic, macrobiotic, and integrative medicine and nutrition.

RECOMMENDED READING

Esko, Edward. *Alzheimer's: The Macrobiotic Approach.* IMI Press, Lenox, Mass., 2019.

Esko, Edward. *How the Umeboshi Works.* IMI Press, Lenox, Mass., 2019.

Esko, Edward. *Macrobiotic Nutrition.* IMI Press, Lenox, Mass., 2018.

Esko, Edward, Alex Jack, and Bettina Zumdick. *Diabetes: A Whole Foods Plant-Based Approach.* Berkshire Holistic Associates, Becket, Mass., 2016.

Esko, Wendy. *The Big Beautiful Brown Rice Cookbook.* Square One Publishers, Garden City Park, New York, 2013.

Harper, Virginia M. and Tom Monte. *Controlling Crohn's Disease the Natural Way.* New York: Kensington Publishers, 2002.

Jack, Alex and Bettina Zumdick. *Macrobiotic Wellness.* Becket, Mass: Planetary Health, Inc., 2020.

Kushi, Aveline and Wendy Esko. *The Changing Seasons Macrobiotic Cookbook.* Avery Trade, 2003.

Kushi, Aveline and Alex Jack, *Aveline Kushi's Complete Guide to Macrobiotic Cooking.* Time-Warner, New York, New York, 1985.

Kushi, Michio and Marc Van Cauwenberghe, MD. *Macrobiotic Home Remedies: Your Guide to Traditional Healing Techniques.* Square One Publishers, Garden City Park, New York, 2015.

Kushi, Michio and Alex Jack. *The Book of Macrobiotics: The Universal Way of Health and Happiness.* Square One Publishers, Garden City Park, New York. 2012.

Kushi, Michio. *Your Body Never Lies: The Complete Book of Oriental Diagnosis.* Square One Publishers, Garden City Park, New York. 2010.

ENDNOTES

[1] Quoted by Jane E. Brodie, "Babies Know a Little Dirt Is Good for You," *New York Times*, January 26, 2009.

[2] Alanna Collen, *10% Human: How Your Body's Microbes Hold the Key to Health and Happiness*, HarperCollins, 2015, 64.

[3] Ibid.

[4] Ibid.

[5] Gevers, D. et al., "The Treatment-Naïve Microbiome in New Onset Crohn's Disease." *Cell Host Microbe,* March 2014;15(3):382-392.

[6] Quoted by Chris Comish, "Distinct Microbiome Detected in Patients with Crohn's Disease," www.bionews-tx.com, n.d.

[7] Patricia Inacio, Ph.D., "Microbiome Imbalances Can Induce Crohn's Diseases-like Inflammation," IBD News Today, www.ibdnewstoday.com, April 27, 2015.

[8] Ibid.

Printed in Great Britain
by Amazon